# ABOUT THE AUTHOR

Peter Fraser was a bookselle
ering Homœopathy. His wo.
remedies led to an interest in c
resulted in his book The AIDS ₁

Having done work on definii.                  ..nes of the
Realms, he was fascinated by th\     ..reatures and substances that move between the Realms and the dynamic
pictures generated by this movement which both defines
the group and differentiates within it.

# OTHER WORKS BY PETER FRASER

### From Winter Press
The AIDS Miasm: Contemporary Disease and The New Remedies

*The Using Maps and Systems in Homœopathy series*:
Using Realms in Homœopathy
Using Mappa Mundi in Homœopathy
Using Miasms in Homœopathy
Using Philosophy in Homoeopathy
Using Correspondences in Homœopathy
Using Archetypes in Homœopathy
Using Provings in Homœopathy
Casetaking in Homœopathy

*Transformation between the Realms:*
Insects – Escaping the Earth
Spiders – Suspended between Earth and Sky
Snakes – Drawing power from the Underworld
Birds – Seeking the Freedom of the Sky
plus Drugs, Trees and Lacs

### On the Internet at www.hominfo.org
A Supplement to Clarke's Dictionary of Practical Materia Medica
      (an ongoing project).
The full text of many new provings.
Articles and information on Peter's latest research and ideas.

ISBN 987 1874581185                          r1

Cover design by Colin Winter
Printed by Biddles of Kings Lynn

Text and artwork © Winter Press, 2008
Published by Winter Press in 2008

Winter Press
16 Stambourne Way
West Wickham
Kent  BR4 9NF
e: insects@winterpress.net

# Insects

# –

# Escaping the Earth

TRANSFORMATION BETWEEN THE REALMS

by

Peter Fraser

# CONTENTS

# INTRODUCTION

There are two types of symptom in any case. Most symptoms make up what can be seen as the background of the case. These are stable and distinctive and they will lead the prescriber to a group of remedies. Examples of the background are the Miasms, the Botanical and Zoological Families, the Periodic Table, the Realms and the Kingdoms.

It is sometimes possible to find the indicated remedy by cross referencing the various background features of the case. This approach has great appeal as it appears to be ordered and systematic and does not require a detailed knowledge of the remedies. In fact a completely unknown remedy can be prescribed purely on its relationship to other known remedies. However, this approach is not as easy to work with as it may seem as distinctions are subtle and the slightest misunderstanding in classifying any aspect of the case will lead to the wrong remedy.

The background in the case will usually lead to a group of remedies and it is differentiating within the group and finding the specific group member indicated in the case that is the most difficult part. Although other backgrounds do differentiate somewhat there is usually a correspondence between different backgrounds. Many remedies that are of the Sea Realm are also Phelgmatic in nature and so knowing that a case is both of the

Sea and Phlegmatic is not very helpful.

The foreground is the place in a case where there is dynamic energy and movement. It is the place where the patient becomes animated and where the symptoms are changing and contradictory. This is the place that restricts, that prevents the patient from moving on and growing but it is also the place through which they will move and grow. This is perhaps the most distinctive feature of the foreground of the case, it is as positive as it is negative and it is as healing as it is destructive. It is also unusual, individualistic and characteristic. No one else expresses it in quite the same way and for no one else would it quite make sense in the way it does for the patient. It is also something that appears in different aspects of the case but with the same distinctive quality. The foreground is what Hahnemann refers to as the totality of the characteristic symptoms.

Finding the foreground in a case gives you a deep insight into the patient and without understanding this aspect of their life it is very difficult to understand the case and to discover what it is that is to be cured.

Finding the foreground features in a case requires attention to the patient's way of expressing him or herself and of describing his or her symptoms. The key indicators are animation and contradiction and wherever either of these appear in a case they need to be pursued because here will be found the information that allows an accurate differentiation between the group of background remedies. Animation is important because it indicates that the things under discussion are dynamic and alive for the patient. Contradiction is important because the path to illness and the path to healing are the same just as the symptoms of the disease and of its cure are the same.

The same process that is involved in finding the foreground features of a case is involved in finding the foreground features of a remedy. Again animation and contradiction are the key indicators of foreground symptoms. This is why it is important to study remedies from the provings as all too often these are lost in secondary materia medica.

In some classes of remedy there is at least one point of dynamism and change that is the same for all the group but which the individual remedies each handle in slightly different ways. Each remedy has different issues that dominate the same dynamic process. One of the clearest points of this dynamis is when there is movement from one Realm to another. The Birds, Trees and Insects all involve movement from the Earth to the Sky. The Snakes and Drugs move between the Earth and the Underworld. Since this movement is so important and so dynamic it will be where the dynamic foreground of the remedy is expressed.

Through understanding the way in which each individual remedy handles this point of transformation it is relatively straight forward to differentiate between the members of the group.

# INSECTS – ESCAPING THE EARTH

◇◇◇◇◇◇◇◇◇◇◇◇◇◇◇◇◇◇◇◇◇◇◇◇◇◇◇◇◇◇◇◇◇◇◇◇◇◇◇◇◇◇◇◇◇◇◇◇◇◇◇◇◇◇◇◇◇◇◇◇◇◇◇◇◇◇◇◇

Insects are the largest class of animals with some 800,000 species described and possibly a far greater number that have not yet been found. For every human on earth there are something like a billion insects. They range from stick insects a foot long and moths with a 12 inch wingspan to many tiny species one hundredth of an inch long. They are generally among the most developed of the invertebrates. The evolution of the insects allowed for the co-evolution of the angiosperms, the flowering plants that make up the majority of plant species. Many insects live off the nectar that they receive from plants in return for pollination. However, they can also be parasites and the parasites of parasites. Many feed on dung or decaying material and without them the ecosystem would be overwhelmed with partially decayed organic material in a matter of weeks. The ecology of the planet is dependent on the activities of insects.

What exactly constitutes an insect is not clearly defined. Sometimes all the six-legged hexapods are regarded as insects; sometimes only those which fly or have flying ancestors. As only the latter group are used in homœopathy the question is fairly unimportant to us.

The chief features of insects are that they fly; that they develop from juvenile forms that are often very different from the imago (adult); that they breed prolifically; and that many of them are social animals. By no means do all insects have all these features but they are the features of the insects as a whole and they seem to be found, at least to some degree, as features in all Insect remedies, even those made from insects that do not express all of them in their current physical forms.

The insects and the birds are the only classes of animal that have established the ability to fly as a property of most of their species and so a property of the class as a whole. Some mammals, particularly the bats, some snakes and lizards and even some fish have the ability to fly or at least to glide but they are all exceptional within their class, with insects and birds the inability to fly is the exception.

Almost all insects undergo some form of transformation from their larval form to the adult form. Some are holometabolous and undergo a pupal stage in which they change, often into a completely different form. Others are hemimetabolous and undergo a series of changes through a number of larval stages, called instars, as they shed their exoskeletons, each one a little more like the adult form. The common pattern involves a flightless larval stage and a winged imago. The appearance and feeding behaviour of the two forms can be completely different. The caterpillar and the butterfly being the most powerful expression of this.

Insects use a wide range of reproductive strategies. The adults are usually involved in sexual reproduction, though there are species that reproduce sexually at the larval stage. Some insects use a degree of parthogenesis, with the child a clone of the mother. Usually when this happens sexual and asexual reproduction are found in alternating generations but there are species that are only known to reproduce asexually. Sometimes the larvae reproduce asexually and only some generations reach maturity and then reproduce sexually. Insects are also often involved in the sexual behaviour of plants. Some plants, most notably species of orchid, pose as sexually available insects to attract mates who will pollinate them.

Although it is not entirely the norm for insects, there are many that are social. They can establish enormous colonies with many different forms each suited to its particular role in the society. Behaviour in such societies is often controlled by complicated systems of chemical signals. The result is that the colony behaves as if it is a single autonomous organism. Even insects that do not form social colonies often live in some sort of looser social arrangement. Many also form complicated parasitic or symbiotic relationships with other insects, plants and animals.

Insects are generally industrious. The main form found in any of the social insects is the worker. Generally they are able to do enormous amounts of work, whether it be creative or destructive. They can eat their way through vast quantities of whatever it is that they eat and they can create substantial and architecturally impressive nests or colonies or tiny cocoons of the finest silk.

The insects are the things in this world for which transformation is both qualitatively and quantitatively the most powerful and the most dramatic. Many of them change completely in form and, on the whole, the transformation is from something earthbound and repulsive to something much more beautiful that is free to move through the air.

Like the Birds the Insects move from the Earth into the Sky but there are substantial differences in what this means for them. The most important difference is a subtle one but it is the one from which the others spring. It is that the Insects are escaping from the Earth while the Birds are moving into the freedom of the Sky.

The aspiration of the Birds, the desire and need for freedom and the desolation at being trapped and denied freedom is the most important thing to them. For the Insects where they are going is unimportant it is the shame or dirt from which they are escaping that matters to them.

The Earthly Realm from which the Birds are escaping is unimportant to them, it is what they are leaving behind. You will find a range of similar origins to the feeling of being trapped in all the Bird remedies and where it comes from will not differentiate the remedies. The Sky Realm is also no help in differentiating the remedies. Freedom is free, any attempt to define it immediately puts restrictions on it and so would make it no longer free. The Bird remedies are defined by the thing which prevents them from reaching the Realm of the Sky and the freedom it offers. It will be the same thing that allows them transformation and freedom but in a pathological state they will see it primarily as the thing that thwarts them.

For the Insects the Realm of the Sky, the place to which they are escaping is not important. The thing that defines it for them is that it is not the Earthly Realm where they are subject to the restriction of society and to dirt and shame. The Sky is for them, if they consider it at all, a fantasy place where they are not subject to the things that they must face on Earth. The things from which they are escaping are also not differentiated. There are many and varied things that they wish to escape but these are not individualised to any remedy. It is not these things but the feelings that they engender that are important and these feelings are similar for all the remedies.

The differentiation lies in the way in which they escape the Earth. Again this is different from the Birds where it is what stops them that is important while for the Insects it is what they can or can't do that matters. It is about the way in which they apply their industriousness and the way in which they transform from earthbound beings into ones that have the freedom of the Sky.

The Birds inherently have the apparatus with which they reach the Sky. Chicks need to mature before they can fledge but that is a straightforward and normal process. The flightless birds, which include the remedies: Ostrich, Penguin and Roadrunner, have found other means by which they obtain freedom, whether it be through running or through movement in the water, they therefore no longer have need of flight and the fact that they have lost the power is no disability and does not matter to them.

The Insects are not born in the form that is able to leave the Earth and move into the Sky. They must work, usually through several larval stages and then through a transformative pupal stage and for some, like many parasitic wasps through several generations, before they attain the form and characteristics that allow flight. They have to work hard at this and it takes a great deal of energy which is why many larvae are such prodigious eaters. It is their energy and industriousness that eventually promises them their freedom.

Many species of insect, especially among the Hymenoptera, are social animals. These are ones in which the individuals have specific and different roles. The social unit acts as an entity and the individual plays a role as part of the whole to which its own interests often have to be sacrificed. The individual may not itself achieve freedom but must strive that the group as a whole can. The activities of the individual are regulated by the complicated interaction of many different hormones and pheromones.

# INSECT REMEDIES IN GENERAL

The key indicator for the Insect remedies is there industrious-ness. It is through the work that they do that are able to progress and so their work is always important to them in some way. They will put all their energies into their work and it will be among the ways that they gauge their success. This could be a little misleading as it is the work itself that is important rather than the concomitants such as success, power and recognition. Though in the individual Insect remedies the importance of some of these rewards can be pronounced and thus a point of differentiation. In non insect remedies the things that come from work are often more important than the work itself.

The Insect remedies will also bring a work pattern and ethic to whatever they do. This means that they do things in a business like manner, even things where this is not appropriate and so they can appear to be unemotional, structured and fastidious, especially in personal relationships. They are better for activity and for work rather than just any activity. They are restless and are often unable to rest or to settle into a calm or meditative state. However, their restlessness can become unproductive, just buzzing around getting nothing done.

It is only through effort that they are able to achieve and it is only through achievement that they are able to gain validation for who they are and what they do. It is achievement rather than success that is important to them and not so much for its own sake or even for what it brings but because it validates their work and their effort. The other side of this can be that in spite of the work they do and the effort they make they do not achieve as much as they feel they ought and they find this very depressing.

One of the areas that the Insect remedies can direct their energies is into benevolence. They can be working for the good of the family or the group rather than just for themselves. They feel that helping others can be very worthwhile and this is another way of validating the work that they do. However, they also feel that others should reciprocate and should help them and they are disappointed that they seem to give much more than they receive in the way of help and support from the people around them.

The Insect needs to metamorphosize, to transform, in order to be able to do what he or she needs to do. It is not enough for them just to grow or develop or learn. The way that they are is not sufficient to achieve their objectives and needs. They feel that they need to be a different person and in a different situation in order to be able to move on. They might need to change their environment or the company they keep. They might feel they need to learn something more or to gain new skills or to achieve some sort of qualification. At the same time there is a reluctance to take the necessary steps and a feeling that in changing they will lose something of what they already have.

There can be a paradox arising from the attitude to transformation in that they must work and through work achieve something in order to transform but they also feel that they cannot truly achieve through their work until they have transformed. They feel this puts them in an impossible situation that seems to have no resolution and so they despair of ever being able to make the necessary transformation.

Exhaustion is found throughout the Insect remedies. It is a physical exhaustion that comes primarily from too much activity. One of the patterns found in many of the provings is a sense of physical exhaustion that comes with a sense of mental energy and alertness. It is as if the body can't keep up with mind. There are so many things to be done and so many ideas to be explored that the body runs out of energy long before they are done. This is further exacerbated by the fruitless nature of much of the activity which results in a great deal more energy being expended than is entirely necessary.

There is much laziness, ennui and a lack of motivation in the Insect remedies. Some of this follows from the exhaustion, some of it comes out of a sense of despair that there is no progress and that enormous effort never actually produces results. However, there is also an innate laziness and a desire to do nothing. The restlessness also means that they are continually looking for something new and become bored very easily with having to do the same thing.

The Earthly Realm is to do with the material world and with possessions and wealth and these things are important to the Insect remedies. They have concerns about money, worry about poverty and have a tendency to spend more than they can afford. They like to have things that are of value and particularly things that are a little bit ostentatious. Though at the same time there is an understanding that possessions and materialism hold them to the Earth and hinder their spiritual transformation.

The Insect remedies have a desire to be seen, to be looked at and to be recognized. It is partly through their work that they seek recognition but there is also a strong personal dimension. They want to look good and to be well dressed. The things that they wear are bright and colourful and they will be noticed. They are vain and want to look at themselves in the mirror. They spend too much money and particularly on clothes and jewellery, hair is a particular focus of this aspect of the remedies. They want their hair to look good and feel that it is a very important part of how they look. Almost all the Insect remedies also have some symptoms around hair falling out, alopecia and a fear of losing their hair.

There is in the Insect remedies a duality. This is not the same as a contrary or a polarity. A duality is when there are two opposite things that are very important but which are entirely incompatible. In a duality there is no possibility of compromise and no sense of a place in between where both aspects are accepted in some way. It is one or the other. A common expression of duality is in the phrase "seeing things in black and white", where the very concept of grey is excluded. The Insect remedies do see things in black and white and they have a similar attitude to lightness and darkness, good and evil, being present and not being there and to gender and sexual orientation. This aspect of the Insects together with their business like attitude to things makes them easy to confuse with the Minerals: black and white attitudes and a structured approach to everything being generally accepted as key indicators of a Mineral remedy.

However, the "black and white" attitudes found in the two groups are significantly different. In the Minerals we find the most primitive understanding of the world. It is an understanding that does not encompass complexity and so has no space for the grey areas. To understand the either/or is both enough for them and all they are able to comprehend. For the Insects the black and white attitude is an aspect of their duality and is a much more complex thing. Because many insects are able to be present in two very different and often contradictory forms: the larva and the imago, the caterpillar and the butterfly, their understanding of the world tends to also take two separate and often contradictory forms. Because both forms cannot coexist and because, just as their transformation is often sudden and complete and does not include intermediate states, they do not work well with change that involves smooth development and have difficulty understanding compromise and grey areas. They therefore enter into the state of duality the two contradictory states are either alternated between or held together in a state

13

of active conflict.

A good example of the comparison can be seen in the confusion of sexual identity. This is found in the Minerals Hydrogen and Iridium. In Hydrogen the spirit of the patient is unsure about coming to Earth, about manifesting at all. Decisions that follow later, such as in what gender to manifest are addressed to an even lesser degree and so the patient is unsure as to what gender they are. It does not generally involve deep conflict it is merely an uncertainty, a confusion. Iridium is concerned with boundaries and with establishing difference and boundary. The Iridium patient is uncertain as to where the boundary lies between masculine and feminine and their struggle is to define and understand that boundary. In the minerals it is confusion that is apparent. There is not so much conflict and what there is arises from confusion.

In the Insects the confusion of sexual identity is most strongly expressed in the Housefly and this is the remedy in the repertory, but it is a conflict this is, I think, to be found in the Insects in general. It is much more a conflict than just a confusion. Both masculine and feminine elements are strong in them but they are unable to integrate them into some sort of compromise that allows an expression of both. They feel that it must be a situation in which it is either one or the other. They therefore tend to create a duality where the two are expressed separately or in alternation and where there is a painful conflict between them. Sexual orientation can become an issue in the same way. They may have bisexual tendencies but the concept of an intermediate, compromised state such as bisexuality is anathema to them and they will be unable to adapt to it. Rather they will set up a situation where both homosexuality and heterosexuality are expressed but are in conflict with each other.

This situation may be an internal one but it can also be externalized into the way that they are perceived by others. In particular their appearance or behaviour may cause others to wonder if they are homosexual or to make homosexual advances to them and they find this very disturbing.

Confusion of various types is found in many of the Insect remedies. There can be considerable confusion arising out of their exhaustion, although on the whole it is a physical exhaustion and the mind often remains clear. The most commonly expressed confusion is around expression either in speaking or in writing: mixing up letters or words. Forgetfulness is also common in the remedies, particularly for names and in several provings the names of close friends could not be remembered.

The Insect remedies have a tremendous sensitivity. It is a sensitivity to the environment in particular. Some or all of the senses are likely to be more sensitive and acute. This sensitivity relates to their tendency to irritate and be irritated. All of the senses, particularly hearing, are likely to be on edge and the least sound will cause irritation and irritability.

The Insects are what they eat, generally more so than other animals. The general naming of insects often involves the naming of the type of insect and of the plant that it infests and consumes. Several remedies are defined in this way, not just by the insect but also by the plant they live and feed on. These include the Oak Gall Wasp: Galla querus robur, the Aphid: Aphis chenopodii glauci and the Cochineal: Coccus cacti. Many insects are poisonous and more often that not they accumulate the toxins found in the plants they feed on rather than creating their own. In the same way the symptomolgy of the plant is often grafted on to the picture of the insect. Coccus cacti for example has heart symptomology that is clearly similar to the symptoms found in Cactus.

They can be sensitive to the feelings of other people but this is much less strong than it is in the Birds, the Spiders or the Snakes. It is rather that they are sensitive to the presence of people as part of the environment. They feel vulnerable, not only to physical attack but also psychically. It is as if people are able to psychically invade their space and so to harm them.

Some of this feeling may be related to the importance of

social interaction to the remedies. Many insects live their lives as part of a colony that acts as if it were a single organism. The individual is often under the control of the colony and not only its development but also its behaviour is controlled by the pheromones and chemical signals that come from the rest of the colony. The struggle for individuality and recognition and the desire to conform are one of the important dualities and contraries to be found in the Insect remedies. The need for company and the desire to be alone are likewise common, contrary and dynamic in many of the Insect remedies.

Sexuality is an important aspect of these remedies. The insects are generally extremely prolific, reproducing quickly and in great numbers. Many insects have developed very specialized and complicated mating patterns and rituals. Some social insects have only one breeding female and the other females become infertile workers. Some insects use primarily asexual reproduction or alternate between sexual and asexual generations. On the whole there is an urgency to their sexuality. Some of the larval, nymph and pupal stages of the insect lifecycle may be very long but the adult stage tends to be very short and so they need to mate and lay eggs as quickly as possible on reaching maturity. The sexual behaviour of insects and of the flowering plants are often deeply intertwined. The plants often require insects to pollinate them and this is often integrated into the sexual behaviour of the insect. This has come about through a long history of co-evolution and many plants and insects have become completely specific to each other. Each species of Ficus (fig trees) has a single specific species of wasp that is required to fertilise it and whose sexual behaviour requires that particular fig. Other insects live on animals and often eat from the animal, particularly by drinking blood. For many this is tied into their sexual and reproductive behaviour. The female mosquito must have one blood meal before she is able to lay her eggs.

The Insect remedies are often very sexual with sexual behaviour, promiscuity and many sexual dreams. The concern with appearance and with being noticed already mentioned often has a sexual element to it. Sexual perversion came up in many provings, particularly in the dreams, and it seems to be an important factor in these remedies. In some ways this conflates the importance of sexuality with the insect feelings of dirtiness, shame and disgust.

The Insects are escaping from the Earth and their view of it is of dirt and shame. Many insects, especially in their larval forms, are among the creatures most likely to arouse deep disgust and hatred in us. Cockroaches, maggots, fleas and lice are all considered indicators of dirt and many insects are common vectors for disease. There are in the Insect remedies diverse attitudes to dirt and disease but in some way they are usually important. Cleaning and tidying are therefore a common expression of their industriousness. There is a tendency to notice dirt and foulness around them and dreams often involve dirt, decay and shit. The most important expression of this is internalised, the patient feels that they are dirty and that people react to them with disgust. A feeling of shame and of being despised is therefore common in the Insect remedies.

The Insect remedies escape the Earth by flying. Many insects are now either wingless or flightless but in evolutionary terms all of the Pterygota are descended from winged ancestors. If they have lost their wings or the ability to fly it is because they no longer have any need for them. The ability to fly is not something that they strive or yearn for. However, most larval and nymph forms do not fly. Usually they must develop and transform before they are granted their wings. A sense of lightness and flying and dreams of floating or flying are to be found in many of the remedies, but the opposing feeling of heaviness and of being trapped and held back or held down are also representative of the remedies.

Insects breed very quickly and prolifically but they also form the diet of many other species and are consumed in great numbers. The sense of vulnerability is very strong in almost all Insect remedies and all of them have dreams of war, violence and of being attacked.

The Earthy nature of the remedies is expressed in the main physical symptoms. This can be clearly seen in a comparison with the Spider remedies. The Spiders live on a nervous energy and so do not express the symptoms we expect to accompany restlessness and high levels of activity. The Insects work on a more physical plane and so very much express the symptoms that normally go along with excessive activity. They are physically tired while mentally alert, they have great appetite and are generally hot.

Restlessness, irritability and anxiety are almost always found together. They are physical, mental and emotional expressions of the same underlying disquiet and this is no less true in the Insect remedies where physical restlessness and irritability are matched by a feeling, often insubstantial, of anxiety.

The Insect remedies generally have a strong appetite and are constantly looking for the food to sustain their activity. There can be a loss of appetite but on the whole appetite is increased. It tends not to be a discriminating appetite, so it is canine or ravenous and they will eat anything. If there are desires expressed they are for energy foods, carbohydrates and particularly sugars. It is more likely to be a capricious appetite in which they do not know quite what they want. They are often very hungry but feel full after eating only a little.

The expending of energy in activity tends to create heat and excess heat is a common part of the Insect pictures. There is general heat and especially flushes of heat, indicating that they might be useful at the climacteric.

The pains found in Insect remedies are characteristically burning and this is perhaps one of the consistent indicators for Insect remedies. Because they are already overheated they are usually worse for heat and they like open air and feel better for it even when they are cold. The other common pains are pricking, pinching and stabbing.

The way that the heat and burning are expressed varies from remedy to remedy and can be a differentiating factor. So in Cantharis it leads to blistering while in Apis it is watery and linked to oedema. In Culex it is irritating and more like urticaria.

Irritation and sensitivity are general concomitants of heat, as opposed to numbness which usually accompanies coldness. Irritation and irritability are found throughout the Insects but there is also the other side of this in that they can be extremely irritating to those around them.

Inflammation, irritation, urging and burning pain in the urinary organs are pretty well universal in the Insect remedies and they are often associated with an irritation and excitement of the gentitals. There is also urging and incomplete evacuation of the rectum.

Swelling and constriction in the throat appears in almost all the remedies and in many of them there is swelling of the glands in the neck and they can be remedies for mumps. The voice is hoarse and often lost.

# TAXONOMY

The taxonomy of the insects is complicated and, as with all taxonomy, is in a state of flux as new techniques, particularly the analysis of DNA, lead to a clearer and deeper understanding about the relationships between species.

Insects are part of the animal kingdom. They are found in the Phylum of Arthropods, which are primarily defined by their exoskeleton and which include the Crustaceans, the Myriapods and the Arachnids. The subphylum Hexapoda includes the the four orders of the primitive Apterygota the Protura, a group of very tiny, blind insects; the Diplura, the two pronged bristletails; the Collembola, that includes the springtails and the Thysanura, that includes the silverfish. These are sometimes classed as part of the Insecta though other taxonomists include only the Pterygota, the insects that are winged or that have winged ancestors.

There are twenty seven orders of insects of which eleven have representatives in the materia medica.

The sixteen orders not represented are on the whole smaller and less important. However, it would be interesting to have information about some of these including the Ephemeroptera, the mayflies; the Phasmida, the stick insects; the Dermaptera, the earwigs; and the Isoptera, the termites.

The information on the remedies that we do know is of varying quantity and quality. Apis and Cantharis are well known classical remedies, but even with them we have more of an acute picture and not much of a deeper understanding of the mental and emotional state. Nearly a dozen insect remedies have been proved over the last decade and for most of them we have an extensive proving picture but not much clinical experience. There are nearly the same number again for which we have minimal information but some indication of how they might be useful.

The remedies discussed here, though in varying depth, are as follows:

Odonata, the dragonflies and damselflies;
Enallagma carunuclatum          Damselfly

Blattaria (or Blattodea), the cockroaches;
Blatta orientalis          Asian Cockroach
Blatta occidentalis          American Cockroach

Mantodea, the mantids;
Mantis religiosa  Praying Mantis

Orthoptera, the grasshoppers, locusts and crickets;
Schistocerca gregaria  Plague Locust

Phthiraptera, the bird lice and true lice;
Pediculus capitis          Head Louse

Hemiptera, the bugs
Aphis chenopodii glauci          Aphid
Cimex lectularius          Bedbug
Coccus cacti          Cochineal

Coleoptera, the beetles;
Cantharis vesicatoria          Spanish Fly
Coccinella septempunctata          Ladybird
Doryphora decemlineata          Colorado Beetle
Lamprohiza splendidula          Firefly

Hymenoptera, the ants, bees, wasps, and hornets;
Apis mellifica          Honey Bee
Vespa vulgaris          Wasp
Cynips calicis (Galla quercina ruber) Oak Gall Wasp
Formica rufa          Ant

Siphonaptera, the fleas;
Pulex irritans          Human Flea

Diptera, the mosquitoes, gnats, and true flies;
Culex musca          Mosquito
Musca domestica          Housefly

Lepidoptera, the butterflies and moths;
Bombyx processionea          Procession Moth
Inachis io          Peacock Butterfly
Lomonia obliqua          (Lepidoptera saturniidae)
Pieris brassicae          Large Cabbage White Butterfly
Limenitis bredowii californica  California Sister Butterfly

# REPERTORIZING

Using the repertory with the Insect remedies is very difficult. Many of the new remedies have not been added yet and most of the old ones are very incomplete.

There is also no representative remedy that gives a good indication that an Insect might be needed in the way that Lachesis does for the Snakes, Falco for the Birds or Tarentula for the Spiders. It is therefore necessary to be able to recognize the Insect remedies even when they do not appear strongly in a repertorization.

Apis and Cantharis are well represented in the repertory although mostly in therapeutic terms and the mind symptoms are fairly restricted.

Coccus cacti and Formica rufa have good representation but again not much of a mind picture.

Cimex, Aphis, Vespa, Doryphora, Pediculus all have some representation but limited picture. Inachio io, though new, has about the same level of representation.

Limenitis bredowii californica, Galla quercus, Musca domestica have all been added to the repertory recently. Although they have the same number of rubrics as the last group their mental pictures are much clearer and they have fewer physicals.

Mantis, Enallagma, Schistocerca, Blatta, Lomonia, Culex, Coccinaella and Lamprohiza all have extensive new provings that have not yet been added to the repertory. Pieris and Inachio are in the repertory but the provings are not available in English.

The other remedies are very poorly represented at this time.

# FAMILIES

⬧⬧⬧⬧⬧⬧⬧⬧⬧⬧⬧⬧⬧⬧⬧⬧⬧⬧⬧⬧⬧

Just as Insects have qualities of the Animal Kingdom in general as well as qualities specific to Insects; so each family or order of Insects has general Insect qualities as well as qualities that are specific to that family. From most of the orders we have only a few representatives but it is still worth making a tentative differentiation that can be clarified and expanded as more remedies are proved and we gain more experience.

Ondonata, the dragonflies and damselflies, have a connection to the Snakes and are fearsome predators. Like the Snake remedies they have some degree of clairvoyance and connection with the Underworld.

Orthoptera, the grasshoppers, locusts and crickets, have enormous amounts of pent up energy that has no outlet and so is held in tension or is vented explosively.

Hemiptera, the bugs, are the most cramped and restricted of the Insect remedies.

Coleoptera, the beetles, is the largest family of all insects and indeed of all animals. It is said that if God created everything he must have had an inordinate fondness for beetles. The Coleopatera is the family in which sexuality is most strongly expressed. It is also the family which bears a strong relationship to rabies and the Hydrophobic Miasm and to the Solanaceae family of plants. Although urinary symptoms are strong in all Insects the cystitis of the Coleoptera is the most extreme.

23

Hymenoptera, the ants, bees, wasps, and hornets, is the family in which the social organization is found most clearly. Issues of competition and jealousy and of establishing individuality in the face of pressure to conform are important in this family.

Diptera, the mosquitoes, gnats, and true flies, is the family in which, while the physical transformation occurs, it is not successful on an emotional level and in spite of it they are still trapped in an Earthly world of dirt and shame. The feeling of being taken advantage of is particularly strong in this family.

Lepidotera, the butterflies and moths, is the family which most completely succeeds in the Insect objective of transforming themselves so they can leave the Earth for the Sky. The issues of struggle are less important but they have little understanding of the place they have achieved.

# ENALLAGMA CARUNUCLATUM – DAMSELFLY

The damselfly was proved by Melanie Grimes. There is also a proving of another species by Jeremy Sherr that has yet to be published. Damselflies are in the same family, the Ondonata, as the Dragonfly and are often loosely referred to as dragonflies.

The Damselfly has large eyes that dominate the head. The eyes have up to 30,00 elements and give them excellent, almost 360° vision. They have two pairs of fine membranous wings and a long thin abdomen and they are often very beautiful.

In folklore dragonflies are associated with the Devil. There is also a connection with Snakes. The Welsh name for them is gwas-y-neidr, "adder's servant". In the Southern United States one term for them, "snake doctor", refers to a folk belief that dragonflies follow snakes around and stitch them back together if they are injured.

Dragonflies and damselflies are particularly skilful fliers and are able to hover and perform aerial acrobatics. They can fly in complex patterns of motion that disguise their movement and make them appear stationary to the prey they are approaching. Eggs are laid near water and the naiads are voracious aquatic predators eating the nymphs of other insects and even small fish. The final moult takes place on a plant close to the water and the adult flies away to mature, returning to the water only to mate and lay eggs.

The predatory nature of the dragonflies is perhaps the strongest individuating feature of Damselfly. There is a sense that they are able to wait almost still and then suddenly pounce. There is a sense that they are high up, observing. Although active like all Insects they are unusual in being able to switch into a calm meditative state. Their hunger, which is ravenous and indiscriminate, has a predatory nature to it and when they decide what they want nothing will stop them. Hunger and hunting go together for them. Symptoms are generally better for eating.

The attention to clothing and looks is there as it is in all Insects but in Damselfy there is a stress on looking clean, neat and well groomed rather than just in looking attractive. One prover stressed that she was wearing clothes in unusual combinations. The issues around cleaning, tidying and organizing are all there, though perhaps with a greater ambivalence about them and perhaps a stress on being clean rather than tidy. There were several dreams of people defecating in their underwear.

There is confusion and loss of memory. Confusion is particularly concerned with orientation: backwards and forwards, left and right. There was a feeling of being disoriented and of being unconnected to where they were. Mistakes seem to have a particular emphasis on repetition. Concentration was difficult and particularly moving attention from one thing or task to another.

There is a duality in a desire to hide away and hibernate and a feeling of being more sociable and feeling comfortable and at home in company. Physically being indoors feels restrictive, too hot and suffocating and there is a strong desire to be outside and in the open air.

Damselfly has the same feeling of vulnerability that the other insects do and it is like them extremely sensitive emotionally. However, it takes this emotional sensitivity even further into the realms of clairvoyance.

There is an affinity to the eyes with strong photophobia, blurred peripheral vision, objects appear two dimensional. There is also irritation of the eyes and around the eyes.

The common urge to stool characteristically comes on on standing up. The back ache and discomfort also has a relationship to standing erect and vertical.

The heat is usually expressed in flushes or waves of heat but there is a burning sensation in the mouth and burning of the skin such as on the palms. There is a thirst for cold water and a desire for cold food.

There is a paroxysmal element to the remedy with cramping pains, particularly in the extremities, a paroxysmal cough and yawning.

# BLATTA ORIENTALIS –
# INDIAN COCKROACH

The cockroach is said to have been introduced into the materia medica when a man's asthma miraculously improved and he later found a cockroach had fallen into his teapot. There was a proving in Mumbai in 1995 by Dr Munjal Thakar.

The cockroach is a flightless insect that runs very fast. They are ancient insects virtually unchanged in millions of years and are extremely hardy. They can survive radiation doses 100 times those fatal to humans. They can live without food for a month and without water for a fortnight. If one's head is cut off it continues to live and only dies from a lack of water and food up to ten days later. They are pests causing damage and contamination to food as well as consuming it and they have a very disagreeable odour. Cockroaches contain similar allergens to shellfish and their body parts in the air can cause asthma.

The strongest feature of the cockroach remedy is a sense of indifference and a numbness that was felt throughout. Provers felt they were less likely to get angry or upset and there was a lack of feeling to friends and family members. They felt physically numb and there was also a lack of facial expression.

The provers did not want to talk or interact with other people and were extremely irritable, acting with irritation and anger to anyone who tried to interact with them. They are abrupt and curt but with a feeling of remorse.

The Blatta patient finds transformation and freedom through work and particularly through professional status and respect. They want to excel in what they do and to be a good person, not so much for its own sake but for the respect and even the veneration that it will bring them. This will give them not only worth and status but also identity. They are prevented from achieving this because they tend to use underhand or at least less than admirable methods to attain their ends and they feel incredibly guilty and remorseful about this.

They feel bad and dirty and this is something that they cannot escape. The more they strive to achieve an honourable place the more they have to use dishonourable means.

Work and professional status are very important. They want very much to be noticed, respected and honoured for their work. They want to wear fine clothes and look good so that they look professional and are admired and respected. They desire to be adored and praised but especially in their professional capacity and they show a reciprocal respect and veneration to their teachers. They show a degree of professional jealousy and are prepared to be argumentative and underhand in order to be noticed. Part of this comes out of a feeling of lacking identity and there is a striving to find their identity, particularly professional identity.

There is a desire to be a good person and remorse that they are not. They use deception and the tricks of the trade in order to enhance their professional position, but they feel very badly about it.

Sexually they can be numb and indifferent. However, they can also be completely overwhelmed by sex and particularly by perverse dimensions of sex which are a feature of all the Insect remedies. There can be a sudden sexual excitement with a desire to talk in a vulgar way and a fear that he would lose control and do something terrible to his girlfriend in a sexual way. There was losing control of his sexual thoughts and saying things he had not meant to say. Along with this is a sense of being dirty or bad and great remorse and guilt. There is a very peculiar sexual symptom with sudden sexual desire and a feeling both emotional and physical of already having had sex and having ejaculated.

The feeling of being bad and dirty is widespread and applies both physically and emotionally. The tongue and skin can be described as dirty. And there is an overwhelming feeling of guilt.

It is important to them that things are done in a systematic and organized way. They had to do things right away, could not put them off and could not rest and laze around until everything had been properly done.

The remedy is very sensitive to cold and there is an aggravation from damp and cold and particularly form the mouldy smells of autumn. Taking cold leads to deep bronchitis.

The oppression of the chest is severe and exhausting. The cough is hacking and unproductive and leads to complete exhaustion and profuse cold perspiration without being able to clear the lungs. The patient has to be propped up as lying down would lead to suffocation. They also feel suffocated by clothing, bed clothes and being indoors.

Although very sensitive to cold the patient is very hot and is said to radiate heat. They want to throw off bedclothes, be fanned, undressed, go outside and take a cold bath. Pains are generally burning in nature.

The patient, like the insect, is photophobic and needs to close the eyes in sunlight. They are also nocturnal: feeling sleepy during the day and alert at night.

## BLATTA OCCIDENTALIS –
## AMERICAN COCKROACH

There is some information from a proving by Mure that indicates an affinity to the liver as well as to the lungs. Jaundice and dropsy are the main conditions found in Blatta occidentalis that are not as strongly represented in B. orientalis. There are pricking pains, violent pains in the temples and chest. The urine is very yellow and there is pain in the urethra on urinating. The lung symptoms are found in both and, on the whole, seem to be similar. It is perhaps indicated when there is dropsy and a strong liver involvement in an otherwise B. orientalis case.

## MANTIS RELIGIOSA – PRAYING MANTIS

There was a brief report in Links of a proving of Mantis religiosa by Walter Gluck. The Mantids are related to the cockroaches and are sometimes classed with them. They are large insects that tend to ambush their prey, which can include small mammals and reptiles, and catch them in their spiny forearms which they hold in an attitude of prayer, hence the name. They are experts of disguise, blending into the background to avoid predators and to surprise prey.

The myth of the Praying Mantis is that the female devours the male, not just after mating as do some spiders, but that she bites off the head of the male during sex and that the thorax and abdomen are able to do the job, or in fact become more vigorous in delivering sperm, without the assistance of the head. There is some dispute as to whether this has been seen because observed matings always take place under stressed conditions. In the cases where this behaviour has not been observed the male has had to go through a long and complex courtship ritual in order to persuade the female from feeding mode to mating.

The themes reported from the proving include those of women suppressed by men and of women who are cold, exclusive and unapproachable.

The dreams were of force, brutality and violence, though the dreamer did not find them shocking, of war and escape and dreams of sexual perversion. All of these are common in the Insect remedies.

There is a sensitivity to change of weather and an affinity to the spine and neurological symptoms.

There is great heaviness of the limbs and it is impossible to lie on the side.

Fear was very strong in the proving and there was a fear of not even being able to get through the day.

# SCHISTOCERCA GREGARIA – PLAGUE LOCUST

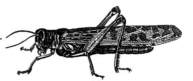

The Locust was proved by Peter Fraser and Misha Norland at the School of Homœopathy in 2007. The Plague Locust has two distinct forms the gregarious and the solitary. The two are different not only in behaviour but also in appearance. The proving was of the gregarious form. When food is scarce not many young survive and those that do remain in the solitary form growing and reproducing slowly. When food is plentiful more survive and repeated contact between individuals (principally the rubbing of bumps on the legs) results in the physical change into the gregarious form which then produces great swarms of not only the imagos (flying adults) but also of the younger non flying forms known as hoppers. This pattern allows the locust to take advantage of years of plenty while lying low in leaner times. It also means that though predators will take them when plentiful no predator will adapt to prey specifically on them.

The swarms of flying locust can cover enormous distances and consume all the vegetation in their path. They have become synonymous with an appetite that eats everything available. At the same time they are preyed on by many creatures including birds, reptiles and mammals and they are the only insects that are kosher and halal and that are commonly eaten by people.

The order of Orthoptera, grasshoppers, locusts, crickets and katydids (bush crickets) include many of the "singing" insects. The sound is made by stridulation, in which the legs are rubbed against the abdomen to produce distinctive sounds.

The structure of insects in this order tends to involve large, powerful rear legs that allow them to jump substantial distances.

The remedy involves a great deal of pent up energy that is held in and cannot be released. They are better for being outside, for exercise, for running and for dancing, where this energy can be allowed to smoothly dissipate. As with most insect remedies they are better for work and activity but in Locust it is specifically because the work allows them to expend some of the energy that is building up. They have the contradiction that going to work recharges and relaxes them while resting at home exhausts them. If it do not have an outlet for their energy they tend to move into a place of explosive release.

This pent up energy often takes the form of sexual energy and frustration with a need for sexual release that overrides all conventional mores and common sense. They must have sex or masturbate immediately in order to dissipate the sexual tension. The physical irritation of the genitals has a strong element of arousal and tension in the Locust.

The common insect irritation will build up and may be released in explosive anger. Physically there is a building of internal pressure and symptoms that echo this, especially a build up of gas released by belching.

Clinical work with Grasshopper indicates that some of the above symptoms are perhaps common to the Orthoptera. There are many symptoms around food and particularly around groups that are probably more specific to the Locust.

The dynamic around being alone and being in the group is particularly important. In the group they feel restricted and suffocated. They are irritated by the people around them and strongly desire to be outside and to be alone. On the other hand being alone is very unsafe and exacerbates the powerful element of fear found in the remedy. If they are alone they are particularly vulnerable but if they have company they are safe. They feel safer outside in the domain of the group than they do inside the home, in their individual domain.

When they feel that they are not being accepted into the group they feel the rejection very deeply. They feel that they are horrible people who will never be liked and cannot be accepted. This is common in Insect remedies but in Locust it is that they are unacceptable to the group more than just to other individuals.

There is a strong need for physical contact and communication, a need to be in touch with people. This contact can, however, also be irritating and it can increase the build up of energy and tension, particularly sexual tension.

The fear in the remedy is deep and irrational. There is a strong fear of the dark, of ghosts of burglars and of sexual predators. The sexual energy and openness seem almost to invite the latter.

The remedy has a more general Syphilitic element. Everything is worse at night and in the dark. There are foul and putrid discharges and odours, foul odours are also perceived or imagined and there is an awareness of dirt and shit. There is excess perspiration and salivation and decay and abscesses of the teeth. There is also paranoia and suspicion, especially that others in the group are talking about them.

The energy and fear give them a feeling of being out of control. Again the group offers a degree of control but at the expense of freedom. They also gain control by cleaning and putting things in order. At its worst the lack of control and the sense of pressure result in a feeling that they are being blown apart into small pieces or that they are just being held together by wires.

There is confusion. This is found in terms of space with getting lost and going the wrong way and in awkwardness and stumbling. It is most pronounced in perception of time. External time was speeded up or slowed down and did not coincide with internal time. Speech and particularly handwriting were affected and an effort was needed to make them clear.

Wherever there is a conflict between the individual and the group confusion of identity is likely. Provers dreamt of their names or their appearance, particularly their hair, being changed.

The pains common to Insect remedies of pricking and stabbing are present but there are also pinching pains and pains in the muscles as of a rope twisted and tightened.

One prover dreamt of lilies and wolves and the pent up sexual energy of Lilium tigrinum and the canine appetite, pack dynamic and menace of the wolf sum up much of the remedy.

# SCHISTOCERCA AMERICANA – AMERICAN DESERT LOCUST

The American Grasshopper was proved by Todd Rowe at The American Medical College of Homeopathy.

The provings of this and the Plague Locust revealed pictures that were almost identical. The issues of energy, often described as a frenzy, and particularly sexual energy; of transformation and change and the physical symptoms were all very similar. In practice the two remedies are probably virtually interchangeable.

If pushed to find a difference the Plague Locust has a more Syphilitic nature with more destructive pathology and a deeper paranoia. The American Desert Locust is perhaps more Tubercular. The attitude to time is slightly different. For S. gregaria the distortion in time is an opportunity it gives them a place to work off their energy and do something useful. For S. americana the distortion puts further pressure on them and they feel they must use every minute and have a particular aversion to wasting time.

## PEDICULUS CAPITIS – HEAD LOUSE

The Head Louse is a small insect that dwells in human hair living off the blood that it sucks from the scalp. It is the scourge of peri-pubescent school children. It is averse to androgens and so is not often found on adult men and is less interested in boys and adult women than it is in girls. The female lays eggs individually gluing them to strands of hair close to the scalp. The empty egg cases remain stuck to the hair and are known as nits. Each female lays about a hundred eggs which mature and start laying their own eggs in about 17 days so an infestation can escalate very quickly. The bite by which they get blood causes itching and irritation. The insect cannot jump and is usually transferred by close contact, they can only live a day or two away from a host. Although it can be a vector for typhus and other fevers in the developed world it is more of a nuisance than anything else.

Just as the insect affects children most so it is the most childlike of the Insect remedies. It has laughing and merriness in a way that the other Insects do not.

It has an aptitude to work, the expressive domain of the Insect remedies, and the usual industriousness. This is particularly expressed in a childlike way with quickness and eagerness, writing with feverish rapidity.

Just as they laugh without cause so their anger and their melancholy can be sudden and causeless.

There is a constriction in the throat and stammering was cured in one prover. Various different noises in the ears were reported. Oedema, fainting and jerking and twitching are all particular. There is violent colic and diarrhoea after eating.

Sexually there are erections without desire and nocturnal emission without amorous dreams.

The usual Insect symptoms of itching, prickling (with horripilation) and irritability both mental and physical, of heat, of falling hair and weariness are all present.

# APHIS CHENOPODII GLAUCI – APHID

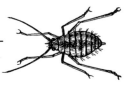

The Aphid is a small insect that feeds on the sap of plants. It often exudes a sticky, sweet liquid called honey dew. Some ants will farm aphids and consume the honeydew. They are a pest to gardeners and farmers and one of the favourite foods of ladybirds.

The remedy is made from aphids that live and feed on the Oak-leaved Goosefoot and undoubtedly shows some of the properties of the Chenopodiaceae, the Goosefoot family, including toothache, colic, convulsions and stupour and paralysis.

The only mental symptom is a general sadness.

It is known for its toothache that is better for perspiration.

There is general dryness. Ineffectual urging of bladder and rectum. Irritation and itching in the urinary tract.

# CIMEX LECTULARIUS – BEDBUG

The bedbug is a small insect often living in the bedding and coming out during sleep to suck blood. It has a strong smelling secretion that it exudes from stink glands. The patient has an odorous perspiration that he himself finds repulsive.

They feel squashed and restricted emotionally and physically. There is restriction and oppression of the chest and of respiration.

The tendons are painfully contracted and contraction and clawing are the most distinctive feature of the remedy.

It has a rage that comes on with fever. It is a remedy for intermittent fevers. The patient would like to crawl inside himself.

There is constipation with hard stools. Urinary incontinence. A hot sensation in the genitals. Shooting pains from vagina to ovary.

37

# COCCUS CACTI –
# COCHINEAL

The Coccus cacti is a small insect that lives and feed on cactus plants. It is collected, dried and crushed to produce cochineal, which was the most important red food colouring and it has been used in cosmetics such as lipstick. It does not have a clear mental picture.

As with many Insects it takes on many characteristics of its host plant and so there are many symptoms close to those of Cactus, especially heart symptoms including sharp pains, pressure and palpitations.

It affects the respiratory organs and is a Tubercular remedy. It also has a whooping cough and weakness and loss of voice. It has haemorrhages.

It is also a remedy for gonorrhoea.

The body is swollen and the skin of the face is cracked.

There are burning pains but also pricking and sticking pains that are close to those of Cactus.

It has the usual irritation, irritability and ill humour. It has constriction of the throat and the sense that the uvula is elongated found in other Insects.

More characteristic are the foreign body sensations such as those of a ball or plug which are found in the throat and in the stomach.

# CANTHARIS VESICATORIA – SPANISH FLY

The Blister Beetle has a long history in medicine and in folklore. It is best know as a powerful aphrodisiac due to the way in which it causes arousal of the genitals though there is always a fine line between excitement and pain. Spanish Fly was used in this way in ancient Rome and the Marquis de Sade ended up in the Bastille when he gave too much to two prostitutes and they were killed by it.

The terpenoid cantharadin is secreted by the male beetle and given to the female who spreads it over the eggs to protect them. It causes inflammation and blistering. When ingested it causes particular inflammation of the urinary tract when it is being excreted hence its stimulation of the genitals.

Blister therapy used the vesicating effect of the insect to create blisters that were hoped would draw poisons out of the body. Cantharadin is still be used in conventional medicine to remove warts, tattoos and molloscum contagiosum.

The remedy was proved by Hahnemann but not included in his materia medica.

The primary use of Cantharis has been in treating second degree burns (i.e. those that blister) and in cystitis and urinary tract infections.

It is the most extreme and wildest of the Insect remedies and takes many Insect features to an extreme place. It is reminiscent of Strammonium, Belladonna and Hyoscymus in its frenzy. It is also like them a Hydrophobic remedy clearly indicated in Rabies.

Like all the Insect remedies it has busyness and activity but because it is so wild there is no control over it and there is no way that it can be productive. Instead they tend to run around in fruitless activity or there activity becomes wild and destructive. They are completely restless and cannot keep still but must move around and also move parts of the body: gesturing or clicking their fingers.

It is also the remedy in which the Insects' sensitivity and irritability are taken to extremes. All tissues but particularly the skin and the mucous membranes are put into a state of absolute sensitivity. The least touch or provocation leads to both great pain and violent over reaction. They are worse from any touch and even from anyone approaching them and are easily offended. There reaction is always excessive and often violent. They scream and behave maniacally from the pain. They can show contempt and cruelty and are cowardly in what they do.

Although sensitive to touch they are better from rubbing. Although their pains are burning they are better from warmth and worse from cold and night. Although worse for being approached and are likely to scream when being approached; they also cry out for help.

The pains are burning and sharp or lancinating and can run along the nerves. There is also a peculiar sensation as if boiling water were being poured over the head. There is a burning thirst. All secretions tend to be increased.

Sexually they are also overwrought with a state of unbearable sexual excitement. They pull at their genitals and masturbate but even having sex does not bring relief from the state of excitement.

The urinary symptoms involve great pain. There is a violent burning pain anywhere in the urinary tract and there is constant urging. Both of these can be before, during and after passing water. Urine is passed drop by drop each one causing terrible pain.

Although Cantharis covers most of the Insect issues it does so in such an extreme manner that it cannot be considered representative of them

# COCCINELLA SEPTEMPUNCTATA – LADYBIRD

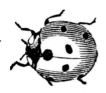

The ladybird with its bright and colourful spotted elytra is much loved, especially by children and with its voracious appetite for garden pests, especially aphids and scale insects, it is also much loved by gardeners. In not causing the usual revulsion felt for insects but instead being regarded as cute and lucky it is unusual. It is associated with the Virgin Mary and its seven spots are said to represent the seven sorrows and seven joys of Mary.

The haemolympha (blood) of the Ladybird is toxic and it is able to bleed it out of its leg joints in order to poison or put off predators. Its bright red colouring acts as a warning of this to prospective predators.

Some physical symptoms of the remedy have been well known but the mental picture has been much enhanced by a proving in Bulgaria by Ekaterina Charmurliyska. The first striking issue in the proving was of accidents and natural disasters, of floods, earthquakes and of houses being demolished. The latter tying in, almost too neatly, to the nursery rhyme. There was great concern for children and animals but also for the homeless, the dispossessed and those, like gypsies, on the fringes of society.

The result of this is a desire to help people and to care for those that need help. There is also a reciprocal desire to be helped and a feeling that people should care for her and make her life easier.

Given that all Insect remedies, and the Beetles in particular, tend to have a strong sexual energy and that the female ladybird is one of the most promiscuous and sexually active creatures in the animal kingdom; a strong sexual element is likely. Lippe reports sexual desire increased and although sex was not strong in the proving there are hints of how it might be important. One female prover was very haughty to her husband, holding out her hand to be kissed in a regal manner. The other side of this was seen in one of the male provers who danced attendance on a female friend, lighting her cigarette and making her feel comfortable.

It seems likely that there is an element of the dominatrix in the remedy and that one partner wants to be treated with excessive respect while the other is excessively attentive.

The provers had a high self esteem and a high degree of self confidence. This is interesting in one of the few well loved insects and is in contrast to almost all other insects which are reviled and feel shame and guilt and have low self esteem. This could come out in aggressive and haughty behaviour. They snap their fingers and point aggressively expecting people to listen and to do as they are told.

The provers had a desire to be beautiful and, as in many other Insects, to buy clothes. One wanted her husband to buy her high heeled boots instead of the books she usually wanted. There was a particular emphasis on colouring the hair and on wearing glittering, sparkly makeup.

The physical symptoms that are most distinctive are the neuralgias in the teeth, mouth and face. They are accompanied by icy cold extremities and profuse salivation. Symptoms tend to jump from side to side and are periodic, usually appearing after an even number of days.

It is a Hydrophobic remedy and all symptoms are worse for seeing bright objects and better for closing the eyes.

It is a remedy for whooping cough and there is a deep, hoarse voice. The uvula feels too long, the tonsils feel swollen and the throat is constricted.

The eyes are swollen and red and it feels as if there is a foreign object under the eyelid. There is also a sensation of sharp splinters in the finger tips.

There is a canine appetite and a desire for milk and sweets and nausea after eating. The breasts feel swollen as if lactating.

All provers felt warmer and it is better for movement and for being outside. The pains are burning and there is a burning pain on urination.

# DORYPHORA DECEMLINEATA – COLORADO BEETLE

The Colorado Potato Beetle is a small yellow beetle with ten brown lines down its back. Its favourite food is the potato but it does eat other Solanaceae such as tomatoes and eggplants.

It is a considerable pest and all the more so because it is highly resistant to toxins and most pesticides have little effect on it.

The picture we have is based on some very small provings and toxicology. It shows some similarity to the other beetles and naturally to the Solanaceae.

The mind symptoms are limited to loquacity, talking about business and irritability so it is not easy to guess what the particular Insect quality of Doryphora might be.

There are the usual urinary symptoms with retention and burning pains. It has been used for the cystitis of pre-pubescents, especially when caused by physical irritation.

The burning pains seem to particularly affect the gastro intestinal tract which is affected from mouth to anus, ending in diarrhoea and bloody, slimy stools. It is a remedy for typhoid fever.

The face is red and bloated, as is the whole body with a bloating that does not pit. The eyes are red, sore, protruding and with dilated pupils.

There is wildness and wild dreams with screaming but there is a great stupor and heaviness about the remedy.

# LAMPROHIZA SPLENDIDULA – FIREFLY

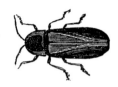

Fireflies are beetles that have developed special organs that use luciferase to combine oxygen and luciferins to create a bright, heatless light. The light can be controlled to produce patterned flashes and is usually part of the process of attracting a mate. However, the larval forms glow when disturbed and the light almost certainly acts in the same way as the ladybird's red elytra to warn of the fact that they, like many beetles, contain toxic chemicals. The remedy was proved by Marty Begin in Toronto.

The distinguishing feature of the Firefly seems to be a sort of naiveté and a feeling that they are just beginning things. They throw themselves into things impulsively and without a full understanding of the consequences. They wanted to try new things: new tastes and new foods, new sex and new work and new ways of living. This was symbolised by the importance of the New Moon.

There is an optimism about the remedy in general but there is also a sense of dread or foreboding. There was a feeling of things about to happen and many of them were terrible, such as plane crashes and being shot. There is often a feeling that things can go either way. Breakdown or breakthrough.

Part of the feeling of things being new and about to happen relates to the Insect theme of rebirth and transformation. It is as if the Firefly is always at the beginning of a new life and they do not know how it will pan out.

They have an anxiety that is felt in the stomach and heart as well as experienced. The anxiety is often about money and work.

Firefly has great energy. It is a bustling, rushing, spinning energy and they not only are better for activity but need to find an outlet for the energy. They will dance, or run, or clean the house. They are restless and their movement is constant and exaggerated.

Like the anxiety, the energy tends to be best expressed in their work. They feel competent and assertive and want to take on their work and get it done. They like to take charge. Provers had long and elaborate dreams particularly about work or travel.

They want to do new things and are bored if they get stuck doing the same old thing. The energy can also end up in antagonism and fighting with everyone.

They want to help and feel good when they are helping and so this is one way that they would like their work to go.

Because they are impulsive they tend to take on too much or to be unprepared for what they have taken on. They can't keep up with everything they have to do and feel they can't get anything done. They feel trapped by this and want to escape the mundane, want to let it all go. They want to be carefree and are torn between responsibilities and being free of them.

The sense of duality is very strong in Firefly. The most fundamental dualities are those of good and evil and of lightness and darkness. The latter of these is something the Firefly physically expresses. Sunshine and moonlight are important and it is often expressed as light breaking through the darkness.

The idea of being there and not being there is also a feature of the physical Firefly, there when light and disappearing when dark, and of the remedy. People disappear and reappear and they feel as if there is something lost or missing. Dualities around obeying the rules and breaking them and around gender are other examples.

There is great sensitivity and they are easily affected by other people's emotions to the extent that provers ended up being consoled by the people who were actually grieving.

They feel vulnerable, fragile and weak. Feel that they can be easily hurt and have a tendency to small injuries and splinters. They don't want to get out of bed as it represents a haven from those who would attack them and they need clothes which they feel act as a boundary and protection both for their sensitivity and their vulnerability.

Like all the Insects there is a desire for attention. They show off and want to be noticed. They are vain and spend time looking at themselves in the mirror.

There is a feeling of numbness and isolation and a desire for company. There is particularly a feeling that they need the help and advice of their friends to counteract some of their impulsiveness.

The Firefly is undoubtedly a magical creature and there is in the remedy a degree of connection to the magical world. Clairvoyance and coincidence were enhanced and some of their sensitivity comes from this. There was also quite a lot of animal energy in the proving.

As in the other beetles there is burning cystitis and a swollen sensation in the throat. There is blistering of the skin, particularly on the hands. The voice is deeper. Breasts tingling as if lactating.

There is a weakness in the back and an aching soreness in the limbs and throughout the body.

There is an affinity to the heart with pains, palpitations and anxiety.

# APIS MELLIFICA – HONEY BEE

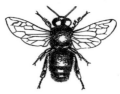

The Honey Bee is a creature of contradiction for us. It is the source of our sweetest foodstuff but it is, of all the creatures that might attack us with poison, the one we are most likely to encounter.

The bee is a social insect and lives in a strictly regimented and almost entirely female society. Each individual has a role to which they are held and there is no other way for them. A single queen takes on the role of breeding, males fertilise the queen once and have absolutely no other role. The majority of the hive are females who have no prospect of breeding.

The remedy is well established in cases of allergic reaction and of oedema but it has a fairly small mental picture.

One of the established and characteristic symptoms of Apis is jealousy. This is often associated with the role of the queen who rules with an iron hand allowing no rivals. It seems to me that the situation is rather of the worker who is not permitted to participate fully in her creative life. She is torn between her role as a worker in the collective and her desire for individuality. She is jealous because she has been denied the full feminine expression which others have as right.

The other characteristic of Apis is an awkwardness which is reported as physical but which Vithoulkas and others extend into the emotional sphere. She, as a worker, feels she is not fully equipped emotionally or physically to fulfil the roles that are involved in a complete life. This is physically manifest in Apis's tendency to abortion, especially in the early months.

The Apis picture is often described as that of the widow who has had her womanly and particularly her sexual outlets removed and is forced to suppress them. In this it corresponds to Conium in the male. However, it could be seen to apply to the nun or the worker bee who has never been able to express herself fully or even had the place to develop the skills and capability to do that.

The worker bee is prevented from developing fully. She has the potential of the queen but because she has been fed a controlled diet she has never fully developed. There is in the remedy the childishness of someone who has never been allowed to grow up. There is foolishness and silliness and laughing over accidents, troubles and misfortunes. The awkwardness is often the gawkiness of the growing child.

While for most Insects work is the means by which they are able to transform and so leave the Earthly Realm; for the Bee the situation is reversed and work is the thing that keeps them tied to the Earth and prevents them from achieving transformation.

The physical symptoms of Apis are violent and sudden and in many ways it relates to Aconite with great fear and presentiment of death. There is great fear of injury and of pain.

Apis is one of the hottest remedies in the materia medica and it is invariably worse for heat in all its symptoms and always better for cool and for cold applications.

The heat of Apis is not a dry one but is waterlogged and it is accompanied by oedematus swellings.

As in the other Insect remedies there is a sensitivity to touch, they overreact to any stimulus. They will scream and cry terribly at the pain of injury or being touched. Burning and stinging pains are felt throughout the remedy.

In the urinary tract there are burning pains and stranguary. In the eyes there is swelling, irritation and photophobia.

# VESPA –
# WASP

The picture we have of the various Vespa remedies is complicated. The only proving we have is of Vespa crabro, the European Hornet. This picture has been conflated with the symptoms of the Wasp, Vespul vulgaris, and with symptoms of the American Hornet, Vespul maculatum, which is not really a hornet but the Bald Faced Yellow Jacket. The symptoms of all three remedies are generally grouped together and are hard to separate. Most symptoms have come from the reports of wasp stings and so there is not much of a mental picture.

While the bee fertilises our plants and provides us with honey to counteract the downside of its sting; the wasp seems to offer us only the sting with none of the compensations. Though hornets are a valuable form of pest control. They kill small insects and neatly butcher them on the spot taking the high protein cuts back to the nest to feed the colony.

The only mental symptoms recorded are great anxiety and insensibility. There is a feeling as if dying that comes on at night.

The pains are as of red hot needles. There is trembling and convulsions and loss of consciousness. Pains in the left ovary.

The other symptoms are all common to the Insect remedies. They include: burning micturation, hoarseness and loss of voice, restlessness, swelling and constriction of the throat, alopecia and inflamation of the eyes.

# CYNIPS CALICIS (GALLA QUERCINA RUBER) – OAK GALL WASP

The remedy is made from a Knopper Oak Gall which is a pathological growth that occurs in place of an acorn. It is caused by the presence of a parasitic wasp and becomes the wasp's home and food source. It is therefore an interaction of tree and insect.

The wasp reproduces sexually and asexually in alternate generations. The male is winged and flies off to fertilise elsewhere but the female in not winged and indolent and so an infestation spreads very slowly. The remedy was proved by Misha Norland in the Czech Republic.

The strongest sensation is one of isolation and of being separated from the world. As if under a thick blanket or behind a thick curtain or a brick wall. There is a feeling of emptiness, as if at a funeral. Also a feeling of homesickness.

There is a feeling of being ostracised and a sense of paranoia that others are talking about them or conspiring against them. They feel like a parasite.

There is also a sense of lightness, of being inflated and of being blown away.

There is crudeness and sexual talk.

The sensitivity and irritability of the Insects is found throughout the remedy.

There are the usual burning pains. Heat radiates from the body yet the skin feels cold. It feels as if there is a cold draft and the tips of the fingers and toes feel cold. Heat and cold tend to alternate.

# FORMICA RUFA – ANT

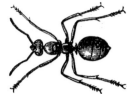

The Ant is another of the social insects with a community arranged around a fertile queen served by infertile female workers. The queen is fertilised in a nuptial flight then returns to earth and rubs off her wings. She spends the rest of her life, which can be fifteen years, producing eggs from the centre of her nest.

The key mental symptom is a happy and exalted mental state that can change suddenly to sadness and depression. There is sudden mortification and grief.

There is a remarkable activity of mind and ability to get on with their work. Everything seems easy to accomplish. They do not get exhausted like other Insect remedies and Formic acid is the only acid which does not feel exhausted.

There is sexual excitement and lewd dreams. There are erections but also the feeling that the genitals have gone to sleep.

Perspiration is profuse but does not relieve in the way it might be expected to.

Irritation of the eyes. Falling of hair. Painful urging to urinate. These are all present but without anything to distinguish them from their presence in other Insect remedies.

The characteristic feature of Formica are the gouty and rheumatic pains in the joints and the wandering pains.

They are worse for cold and damp and better for warmth in contrast to other Hymenoptera.

It is an important remedy for nasal polyps.

## PULEX IRRITANS – HUMAN FLEA

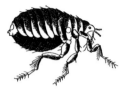

The Human Flea is a very small wingless insect that lives on the blood of mammals preferring humans. It is one of a great number of fleas each of which have evolved to fulfil a niche that is often species specific. Although tiny its rear legs are very powerful and it can jump 200 times its body length. It has a flattened body and a very tough exoskeleton that is not easy to crush and backward facing hairs that allow it to move easily through hair and fur. The bite of the flea usually causes a small raised spot with considerable itching and irritation. In some cases it can cause a more severe allergic reaction.

The remedy does not appear to have been properly proved and the only mind symptoms are the common Insect symptoms of impatience and irritability. However there are a few clear symptoms established through clinical experience.

There are urinary symptoms with frequent urging, burning pain on urination and the flow stops suddenly with great pain.

There is delayed menses with burning in the vagina and profuse, offensive leucorrhoea between menses.

Digestively there is nausea vomiting and bloating.

The eyes feel that they are enlarged and the face appears old and wrinkled.

The heat feels like a glow all over or like being held over steam.

All the discharges, stool, urine, menses and leucorrhoea are offensive and hard to wash out.

# CULEX MUSCA – MOSQUITO

The Mosquito is an enormous pest throughout the world and is the vector of many dangerous diseases but especially of malaria. It was proved by Kent and has had recent provings in India and New Zealand.

The eggs are laid in standing water. The larvae live and feed in the water but come to the surface to breathe. The pupae are unusual in that they are motile, tumbling under water to evade predators and then rising again to the surface. They have a short life cycle that varies by species and is also much slower in cooler temperatures. In the Autumn the fertilised female finds a sheltered place to overwinter, emerging in the Spring to start laying eggs.

They generally feed on nectar but the female mosquito needs a blood meal before she can become fertile and it is her bite and the injection of various substances as she bites that cause a slight allergic reaction with itching, burning and irritability.

Itching, burning and irritability are the keynotes of all the Insect remedies but they are perhaps strongest in Culex. It is found physically all over the body.

Mentally the irritability is extreme and leads to anger and rage that are invariably out of all proportion to the offence caused, which is often trivial. The provers were rude, intolerant, quarrelsome and censorious. If any one invaded their space or offended them in any way their immediate reaction was to fight back and retaliate. Their rudeness and aggressiveness was worse at home than when out and about. Although sentimental about children they find them irritating and are not tolerant of them.

They wish to be the best. This was a word that came through strongly in provings. They wanted to be the best at their work and be the best prover. There is great attention to detail and effort to do things well but it is for recognition and not for its own sake. She wants to gain knowledge, not for its own sake but so she will be the best and this will be recognized.

Similarly she wants to wear the best clothes and the best jewellery so that she will be noticed and recognized for wearing the best. The feeling is that you can easily be underdressed but that there is no such thing as being overdressed. This was echoed in a desire to shop and in spending too much money buying the best things. There is worrying about the hair and concern that it might be falling out.

They feel that they are being taken advantage of and are not going to put up with it but will fight back.

There is also a feeling that she has committed a crime. There were dreams of having committed murder and in reality a feeling that people regarded her as a criminal or thief.

The dreams were full of violence and war and both in the dreams and in reality there was a strong fear of being attacked or murdered. These fears were particularly of being attacked from behind and particularly of being sexually attacked and raped. However, there is a confidence and aggressiveness in the remedy that resulted in the feeling that she would take on whoever attacked her and deal with them.

In spite of the desire for activity Culex is a lazy remedy. There is inertia and procrastination and an unwillingness to get going or to start anything new. The physical exhaustion is most characteristically expressed as heaviness particularly in the limbs and in the eyelids, which can barely be kept open.

Body and mind feel separate. There is also a desire to separate from people and being alone at least ameliorates the irritability. Numbness is found both emotionally and physically, particularly in the mouth and tongue.

They are extremely sensitive but the sensitivity cause them to be irritable and to react aggressively. Nausea is strong in the remedy, particularly after eating, at meal times, at the smell of food or on thinking about food.

There is heat and burning pains but there is also a burning coldness that accompanies the numbness.

Discharges are clear and watery but they are also sticky.

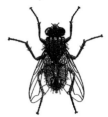

## MUSCA DOMESTICA – HOUSEFLY

The common housefly is one of the most ubiquitous insects, almost always found close to human habitation. The female lays her eggs in decaying material. The eggs hatch in twelve hours and the maggots pupate after 5 or 6 days. The adult flies emerge some days or weeks later, the time being temperature dependent. As 150 eggs are laid by each female and there are a dozen generations in a year the potential number of flies is enormous and only held in check by the large number of predators that feed on them. The larval maggots eat only dead and decaying material. The adults do not eat but use saliva to externally digest food which they then suck up through their proboscis. As they move between decaying and faecal matter and prepared food they are serious vectors for many different diseases. The remedy was proved in New York by Susan Sonz and Robert Stewart.

While the Butterfly represents the Insect that has achieved its aspiration and transformed itself so it can take to the Sky; the Housefly has done everything it should and made the effort. It has undergone the transformation and taken to the air and yet the effort has been in vain for it is still mired in the filth in the dirt and shame of the Earth.

The remedy is as close to shit and garbage as is the fly itself and in the proving images of dirt and filth were powerful in the dreams and in reality. They noticed garbage and dirt. They felt that the remedy was degrading and decomposing in nature. The language used to describe things, particularly themselves, involves words like rotten, crap, oily and dirty.

They feel, as do other Diptera, as if they are being taken advantage of but while the Mosquito will fight back the Fly internalizes it. "I always had to swallow other people's shit." They feel that they help other people but that no one will help them. They do not let things go but nor do they resolve them; thus the image of picking at sores until they bleed, which came to one prover, is particularly descriptive.

Sexuality is very important in the remedy and there is to it an element of perversion. This is true of all the Insects but it is strongest in Musca. Sexual energy and sexual desire were both increased as was a need to masturbate. The feeling in the dreams and in reality was of sexuality that was gross, corrupt, dirty and commercialized. Homophobia and a feeling that homosexuals are corrupt is also there. Confusion of sexual identity is also strongest in Musca and patients are often torn between homosexuality and heterosexuality.

They are better for exercise and desire activity. One prover described exercise as making her insides sing. However, work and career are not as important as they are in many other Insect remedies. Cleaning, on the other hand, which combines activity with a stress on dirt, is even more pronounced in Musca.

There is a sense of having undergone a transformation but it is not as freeing as it should be and there is more of a sense of having to do it again and again. Although there is lightness and flight, particularly in the dreams, the feelings of heaviness, hopelessness, guilt and despair are much stronger.

They are irritable and particularly sensitive to noise and high pitched sounds. They are also aggressive and contemptuous, though they feel badly about it.

They want to be seen and can be provocative but also have a fear of being seen or watched and their feelings of vulnerability are particularly around being observed. There is a compulsive need to buy things and particularly clothes.

It is a fearful and anxious remedy, with a particular anxiety about the family and a fear that they will be hurt.

Physically there is a tendency to herpetic eruptions which were experienced by almost all the provers. One prover experienced a dramatic cure of her long standing rheumatoid arthritis.

Clumsiness, forgetfulness, numbness and a sense of isolation are also all important.

## BOMBYX PROCESSIONEA – PROCESSION MOTH

The caterpillars of the Procession Moth have hairs that cause great irritation. In the remedy there is a sensation that something is being forced under the skin but there is not a clear picture.

## INACHIS IO – PEACOCK BUTTERFLY

There has been a German proving of this remedy and it is well represented in the repertory but I have not seen it yet. It would appear to be more quarrelsome and angry than the California Sister.

## PIERIS BRASSICAE – LARGE CABBAGE WHITE BUTTERFLY

This also was proved in Germany and is in the repertory but I have not been able to study it.

## LOMONIA OBLIQUA –
## (LEPIDOPTERA SATURNIIDAE)

The poison on the hairs of this caterpillar are incredibly toxic and may be the most venomous substance produced in nature. It is an anticoagulent that causes haemorrhage. It was proved in Brazil. In the remedy the most important symptom would seem to be anaesthesia. It is experienced both physically, especially in the lips, and emotionally. There is sexual excitability and great priapism during the night without lascivious dreams. Desire for cold milk. Severe stitching in right abdomen. Increased vital heat; so hot at night that he must sleep naked.

## LIMENITIS BREDOWII CALIFORNICA –
## CALIFORNIA SISTER BUTTERFLY

The California Sister Butterfly is found on the West Coat of the US. It has black and white markings that are said to resemble a nun's habit, hence its name. Like many butterflies it has a large orange spot on each wing that predators might mistake for the eye of a much larger creature. It lays its eggs on oak trees and the caterpillars live off the oak leaves until such time as they pupate. The adults eat fallen fruit and sometimes nectar. They tend to be found close to oak woods and are territorial. There are two generations per year. It was proved by Nancy Herrick in California and is the only proving of a butterfly in English with a substantial mental and emotional picture.

The butterfly is the insect that achieves the insect's objective. It manages to leave the dirty grubby world of the caterpillar and transform into the beautiful airborne butterfly. The Butterfly is Psyche, the free and unlimited soul. A prover described this as a state of emotional freedom and love without hindrance of responsibility and thought.

The Butterfly, because it has reached, or at least does reach, the state of freedom in the Realm of the Sky, is not as concerned with the process of transformation as the other insects are. There are hints and shadows of the process but they are relatively unimportant. The things that are important to the Butterfly are to do with how they feel having reached the Realm of the Sky. This is expressed in several ways.

One is a sense of urgency. The butterfly only has a few days to find and court a mate and to find a place where she can lay her eggs before she dies. There is in the remedy an urgency in everything she does particularly in the area of sexuality. There is strong sexual desire. There are particularly dreams of an orgy and lots of people in bed together. There is an animal sexuality to the remedy.

The other area is in a sense of being thrown into the world without guidance or protection. They feel like a child or adolescent but one whose parents are not there to give them the help that they need. They feel that they need to be helped and taught about this new world. They feel lost in the world, feel like an alien and cannot even tell which side of the street they are on.

They feel terribly vulnerable, that they can be attacked and hurt. Many dreams are of being attacked. There is a sense of danger, so much so that she feels she has to whisper in the morning. Anxiety that something evil had come into the house. They also feel that they wear their emotions on their sleeves and that makes them even more vulnerable.

Whereas the other Insects reach physical exhaustion but are still mentally aware; the Butterfly goes beyond this and both physical and mental faculties become exhausted leaving only the emotional. The mind feels slow as if its gears are mired in a viscous liquid. Just wants to think emotional thoughts. Doesn't want to think but to connect only to the emotional and psychic realms.

The material sphere feels gross and they do not want to be

there, rather they want to move on completely. She wants to go into a mindless state but not to sleep or to be without intelligence.

On the other hand the world is felt viscerally and deeply. There is an extreme physicality, people and things feel smooth. There is compassion, a loving feeling and a spontaneous feeling of pleasure.

Duality is important as in a dream where she was a dark haired man fighting with a blond man. He plays unfair and she attacks him with animal ferocity.

The nose is stuffed up but there can also be a great sensitivity to smell. When I smell my wife and family it is a savouring that permeates through my being.

There is a desire for and they are better for the open air. There are pressing headaches and the eyes feel compacted and pressed in.

Face hot flushed and burning. Heart palpitations. Burning at the close of urination.